Copyright © 2022 by Monica Dimitrios

All rights reserved. No part of this publication may be reproduced, distributed, or transmitted in any form or by any means, including photocopying, recording, or other electronic or mechanical methods, without the prior written permission of the publisher, except in the case of brief quotations embodied in critical reviews and certain other noncommercial uses permitted by copyright law.

Table of Contents

ADRENAL FATIGUE DIET

The adrenal fatigue diet is a food-based approach to improving stress on the adrenal glands. Your adrenal glands are located above your kidneys. They produce hormones that help your body to burn fat and protein, regulate sugar and blood pressure, and respond to stress.

ADRENAL FATIGUE DIET RECIPES

1. Vegan Aquafaba Mayonnaise

Prep Time: 5 mins

Total Time: 5 mins

Servings: 6

Ingredients

- 3 tablespoons aquafaba (liquid from can of chickpeas)
- 1 tablespoon red bell peppers, peeled and cut into 1/2-inch pieces
- 1 tablespoon lemon juice
- 2 teaspoons Dijon mustard
- ½ cup avocado oil
- salt to taste

Directions

1. Combine chickpea liquid, whole chickpeas, lemon juice, and mustard in a tall container. Using an immersion blender, blend on high speed until smooth.
2. Reduce speed to low and slowly drizzle in oil until creamy. Season with salt. Cover and refrigerate for up to 1 week.

Prep Time: 20 mins

Total Time: 55 mins

Servings: 6

Ingredients

- 3 tablespoons olive oil, divided
- 1 small yellow onion, peeled and diced (about 1 cup diced)
- 2 stalks celery, chopped (1/2 cup)
- 4 cloves garlic, peeled and chopped
- 1 medium zucchini, diced (about 2 cups diced, about 10 oz whole)
- 1 pound Pure Farmland Simply Seasoned Plant-Based Protein Starters
- 1 ancho chile in adobo sauce
- 3 tablespoons adobo sauce from can
- 1 teaspoon ground cumin
- 1 teaspoon mild chile powder
- 6 cups low-sodium vegetable broth
- 1 (15 ounce) can yellow hominy, drained
- 2 large bay leaves
- ½ teaspoon dried Mexican oregano
- 1 pinch kosher salt, or more to taste
- To Serve:

- 8 sprigs of cilantro, small stems only, or more as needed
- 1 medium avocado, peeled and diced
- 2 medium radishes, thinly sliced
- 2 medium limes, each cut into 6 wedges
- 2 cups tortilla chips

Directions

1. Heat a large Dutch oven or pot over medium heat. Add 2 tablespoons olive oil, then onion, celery and garlic. Cook 3 minutes, stirring occasionally, then add the zucchini. Cook 5 more minutes, until zucchini is slightly softened, then remove from heat. Transfer vegetables to a plate and reserve.
2. Return pot to medium heat. Add remaining 1 tablespoon olive oil, then Protein Starter. Using a wooden spoon, break apart into pieces about 1/2-inch big. Cook 8 to 10 minutes or until Protein Starter is lightly golden. Add ancho chile, adobo sauce, ground cumin, and chile powder. Cook 2 more minutes, breaking up ancho chile with spoon.
3. Add vegetable broth, hominy, bay leaves, oregano, and reserved vegetable mixture. Bring to a simmer over medium-high heat, then reduce to medium-low heat and cook 10 to 12 minutes or until vegetables are tender. Season with kosher salt, if desired.

4. To serve, top with cilantro leaves, diced avocado, and radishes. Serve with lime wedges and tortilla chips, if desired.

3. Protein-Packed Spicy Vegan Quinoa with Edamame

Prep Time: 15 mins

Total Time: 45 mins

Servings: 8

Ingredients

- 3 ½ cups water
- 2 cups quinoa, rinsed
- 4 teaspoons vegetable bouillon
- 2 ½ cups frozen shelled edamame
- 1 tablespoon olive oil
- 2 sweet onions, chopped
- 2 bell peppers, chopped
- 2 tablespoons minced fresh ginger
- 6 cloves garlic, minced
- ¼ cup reduced-sodium soy sauce
- 2 tablespoons chopped fresh cilantro
- 1 tablespoon hot chile paste

Directions

1. Bring water, quinoa, and vegetable bouillon to a boil in a large pot; stir in edamame, cover, and simmer until quinoa is tender, 15 to 20 minutes.
2. Heat olive oil in a large skillet over medium heat; cook and stir onions and bell peppers until onions

are translucent, about 5 minutes. Add ginger and garlic; cook and stir until fragrant, about 2 minutes. Remove from heat; stir in soy sauce, cilantro, and chile paste.

3. Stir onion mixture into quinoa mixture; simmer, stirring occasionally, until excess broth has been absorbed, about 5 minutes.

Prep Time: 5 mins

Total Time: 35 mins

Servings: 16

Ingredients

- 1 (8 ounce) tub vegan cream cheese
- ⅓ cup vegan butter
- ¾ cup brown sugar
- ½ teaspoon vanilla extract

Directions

1. Bring cream cheese and butter to room temperature, about 30 minutes.
2. Mix butter and brown sugar with an electric mixer until creamy. Add cream cheese and vanilla; mix until completely combined and smooth. Use immediately or refrigerate until needed.

Prep Time: 25 mins

Total Time: 45 mins

Servings: 6

Ingredients

- 3 cups quinoa
- 1 ½ cups water
- ¾ teaspoon adobo seasoning, or more to taste
- 1 tablespoon olive oil, or to taste
- 3 medium sweet potatoes, peeled and chopped
- ¾ cup onion, chopped
- salt and ground black pepper to taste
- 1 ½ cups canned black beans, rinsed
- 3 medium red bell peppers, sliced
- 3 medium avocados, sliced
- 1 tablespoon chopped fresh cilantro, or to taste
- Honey-Lime Dressing:
- 9 tablespoons lime juice
- 6 tablespoons canned coconut milk
- 3 tablespoons water
- 3 tablespoons raw honey
- 1 tablespoon olive oil
- ½ teaspoon salt, or more to taste

Directions

1. Rinse quinoa in a fine mesh strainer and place in a small pot. Add 1 1/2 cups water and bring to a boil. Add 3/4 teaspoon adobo seasoning, lower heat, and simmer until quinoa is tender and water is almost gone, about 15 minutes. Remove from the heat.
2. While the quinoa is cooking, heat 1 tablespoon oil in a skillet over medium heat. Add sweet potatoes and onion and season with salt and pepper. Add more adobo seasoning if desired. Cook over medium heat until sweet potatoes are tender, 10 to 15 minutes. Remove from the heat.
3. Meanwhile, make dressing: whisk lime juice, coconut milk, water, honey, olive oil, and salt together in a bowl. Set aside.
4. Distribute quinoa, sweet potato-onion mixture, black beans, bell peppers, and avocados in 6 bowls. Dress with honey-lime dressing and garnish with cilantro.

Prep Time: 10 mins

Total Time: 50 mins

Servings: 4

Ingredients

- 1 ounce dried porcini mushrooms
- 2 cups boiling water
- 2 tablespoons extra-virgin olive oil
- 1 large shallot, sliced
- 1 teaspoon miso paste
- 1 teaspoon yeast extract
- 8 ounces broccoli, florets separated and stems chopped
- 4 ounces sliced radicchio
- 2 cups water
- 1 cup vegetable broth
- ½ cup hearty red wine
- ¼ teaspoon salt
- 1 cup Italian polenta
- salt and ground black pepper to taste
- 1 tablespoon cornstarch
- 2 tablespoons water

Directions

1. Soak porcini in 2 cups boiling water for at least 10 minutes.
2. At the same time, heat olive oil in a medium Dutch oven over medium heat. Add shallot and slowly saute until soft and juices have been released, 3 to 5 minutes.
3. Remove porcini from the water and use a damp paper towel to remove any grit. Reserve soaking water.
4. Add porcini to the Dutch oven with miso paste and yeast extract. Stir well and reduce heat to a simmer.
5. Add broccoli; put floret heads facing down and stem pieces nestled in so they are touching the bottom of the pot. Layer radicchio slices evenly on top. Pour in wine without disturbing the vegetables. Cover and simmer, occasionally shaking the pan gently, for 10 minutes.
6. Meanwhile, bring 2 cups water, vegetable broth, and salt to a boil. Sprinkle fistfuls of polenta into the boiling liquid while stirring constantly so clumps don't form. Continue to stir in polenta until completely added. Reduce heat to low and cook, stirring often, until polenta is thick and cooked through, about 10 minutes.
7. Strain the reserved soaking water, twice if necessary, to remove any sediment.

8. Pour 1/2 of the soaking water into the Dutch oven with the broccoli. Gently shake the pot and use a wooden spoon to carefully loosen the florets without breaking them apart. Gently fold vegetables over until coated with cooking sauce. Continue to simmer, uncovered, occasionally shaking the pot. Cook until broccoli is tender but still firm to the touch and radicchio is completely wilted. Season with salt and pepper.

9. Pour polenta onto a lightly oiled polenta board and spread it evenly over the board. Use a slotted spoon to gently spoon vegetables over the polenta.

10. Pour remaining soaking water into the Dutch oven and bring to a boil. Make a slurry with the remaining water and cornstarch; pour into the Dutch oven while whisking constantly. Cook until sauce has thickened, 2 to 3 minutes. Pour sauce over the broccoli and polenta or serve on the side.

7. Beyond Beef Vegan Meatballs

Prep Time: 25 mins

Total Time: 1 hr 25 mins

Servings: 8

Ingredients

- 1 (10 ounce) package frozen chopped spinach
- 2 tablespoons water
- 2 (16 ounce) packages Beyond Meat
- plant-based ground
- ¾ cup nutritional yeast
- ¾ cup vegan bread crumbs
- 4 tablespoons tomato paste
- 5 cloves garlic, minced
- 1 tablespoon dried oregano leaves
- 1 tablespoon dried basil leaves
- 1 teaspoon onion powder
- ½ teaspoon salt
- ½ teaspoon ground black pepper
- 4 tablespoons olive oil, divided, or more as needed

Directions

1. Combine frozen spinach and water in a 1-quart microwave-safe casserole dish. Cover and

microwave on high for 5 minutes, stirring halfway through the cooking time. Break up any clumps with a fork and cook for 1 more minute. Transfer to a colander to drain. When cool enough to handle, squeeze small handfuls of spinach to release remaining water and place spinach in a large mixing bowl.

2. Add Beyond Beef, nutritional yeast, bread crumbs, tomato paste, minced garlic, oregano, basil, onion powder, salt, and pepper to the spinach. Mix with your hands until all ingredients are thoroughly combined. Roll into 1 1/4-inch diameter meatballs.

3. Preheat oven to 400 degrees F (200 degrees C). Line a large rimmed baking sheet with parchment paper.

4. Heat 1 tablespoon olive oil over medium heat in a large Dutch oven. Working in batches, add about 12 meatballs and cook, turning often and being careful not to burn, until browned on all sides, about 5 to 7 minutes. Transfer meatballs to the prepared baking sheet, and repeat with remaining batches.

5. Bake in the preheated oven until heated through, 30 to 35 minutes.

6. An instant-read thermometer inserted into the center should read at least 165 degrees F (74 degrees C).

8. Creamy Coconut Curry

Prep Time: 10 mins

Total Time: 25 mins

Servings: 2

Ingredients

- 4 tablespoons coconut butter
- ½ red onion, chopped
- 1 clove garlic, minced
- 1 teaspoon pink Himalayan salt
- ½ teaspoon ground cumin
- ¼ teaspoon ground black pepper
- ¼ teaspoon fennel seeds
- ¼ teaspoon ground coriander
- ¼ teaspoon ground turmeric
- ¼ teaspoon garam masala
- 1 tablespoon cornstarch
- ¼ cup water
- 1 (14 ounce) can cream of coconut
- 4 curry leaves, or more to taste
- ½ teaspoon chili powder
- ½ cup cooked chickpeas
- 2 ounces broccoli florets, chopped
- 4 small heads baby bok choy

Directions

1. Melt coconut butter in a large saucepan over medium heat. Cook and stir onion and garlic using a wooden spoon until translucent and lightly brown in color, 2 to 3 minutes. Season with salt, cumin, pepper, fennel seeds, coriander, turmeric, and garam masala; mix until well incorporated. Stir in corn starch until a creamy paste forms.

2. Slowly mix water into the saucepan to dissolve cornstarch and thicken the mixture. Keep stirring until there are no lumps. Stir in chickpeas and broccoli and briefly cook until just lightly crisp and tender (do not overcook). Mix in coconut cream and curry leaves and cover pan halfway with a lid. Simmer until liquid is reduced and has thickened, 2 to 3 minutes.

3. Remove lid and lower heat to medium-low. Cook and stir until liquid is reduced and curry is thick and creamy, 3 to 5 minutes. Add bok choy and cook until wilted and curry has further reduced, 3 to 5 minutes.

Prep Time: 15 mins

Total Time: 1 hr 5 mins

Servings: 6

Ingredients

- 18 piece (blank)s jumbo pasta shells
- 2 tablespoons olive oil
- 1 (12 ounce) package meatless ground beef substitute
- 1 (15 ounce) can fire-roasted diced tomatoes
- ½ medium onion, diced
- 2 teaspoons minced garlic
- 1 tablespoon Italian seasoning
- salt and ground black pepper to taste
- 3 cups loosely packed fresh spinach
- 1 (15 ounce) container ricotta cheese
- 1 large egg, beaten
- 1 (24 ounce) jar marinara sauce
- 1 cup shredded Parmesan cheese
- 1 cup shredded mozzarella cheese
- ¼ teaspoon Italian seasoning, or to taste

Directions

1. Preheat the oven to 375 degrees F (190 degrees C).

2. Bring a large pot of salted water to a boil. Add shells and cook, stirring occasionally, until tender yet firm to the bite, about 9 minutes.

3. While the shells are cooking, heat olive oil in a large pan or skillet over medium-high heat. Add meatless ground beef and cook and stir until brown, 2 to 3 minutes. Add tomatoes, onion, garlic, 1 tablespoon Italian seasoning, salt, and pepper. Simmer for 2 minutes; add spinach and simmer until spinach is wilted, about 2 minutes more. Taste and adjust salt and pepper if needed. Remove from heat and mix in ricotta cheese and egg until fully incorporated.

4. Pour 1/2 cup marinara sauce into the bottom of a 12-inch cast iron skillet or a 9x13-inch baking dish and spread out with the back of a large spoon.

5. Drain cooked shells. Stuff each with about 1 1/2 tablespoons of the "meat" mixture. Arrange in the skillet or baking dish. Pour remaining marinara over the top. Sprinkle with Parmesan and mozzarella cheeses. Sprinkle with remaining Italian seasoning and more black pepper.

6. Bake in the preheated oven until cheese is golden and bubbly, 35 to 45 minutes.

10. Parsley and Walnut-Crusted Salmon

Prep Time: 15 mins

Total Time: 35 mins

Servings: 6

Ingredients

- 3 tablespoons olive oil
- 1 ½ pounds salmon fillets, cut into 4-ounce portions
- 1 cup chopped packed fresh flat-leaf parsley
- 2 tablespoons lemon juice
- 2 cloves garlic
- ¼ teaspoon salt
- ⅛ teaspoon ground black pepper
- ⅓ cup walnut pieces
- 3 tablespoons chopped toasted walnuts
- 1 lemon, cut into wedges

Directions

1. Preheat the oven to 375 degrees F (190 degrees C). Drizzle 1 tablespoon oil in a 9x13-inch baking dish. Arrange salmon in the dish.
2. Process parsley, lemon juice, garlic, salt, pepper, and remaining 2 tablespoons oil in a food processor until evenly chopped. Add 1/3 cup

walnut pieces; process until combined and walnuts are still a bit chunky. Spread onto salmon.

3. Bake in the preheated oven until salmon flakes easily with a fork, 20 to 25 minutes. Garnish with chopped walnuts and serve with lemon wedges.

11. Pineapple Pie II

Prep Time: 30 mins

Total Time: 30 mins

Servings: 8

Ingredients

- 1 (14 ounce) can sweetened condensed milk
- ½ cup lemon juice
- 1 (20 ounce) can crushed pineapple, drained
- 1 (8 ounce) container frozen whipped topping, thawed
- 1 (9 inch) prepared graham cracker crust

Directions

1. Combine sweetened condensed milk and lemon juice. Stir well. Fold in pineapple and whipped topping. Spoon mix into crust. Chill before serving.

Prep Time: 15 mins

Total Time: 40 mins

Servings: 16

Ingredients

- 1 cup all-purpose flour
- ¼ cup confectioners' sugar
- ¼ cup butter
- 1 cup white sugar
- 2 tablespoons all-purpose flour
- ½ teaspoon baking powder
- 2 large eggs
- 3 tablespoons lemon juice
- 1 tablespoon lemon zest
- ⅓ cup confectioners' sugar for decoration

Directions

1. Preheat the oven to 350 degrees F (175 degrees C).
2. Mix 1 cup flour and 1/4 cup confectioners sugar in a medium bowl. Melt butter and stir into flour mixture. Press evenly into an 8x8-inch baking dish.
3. Bake in the preheated oven for 20 minutes.

4. While crust bakes, make topping: Mix 1 cup white sugar, 2 tablespoons flour, and baking powder in a large bowl. Beat eggs and add to mixture, stirring well. Add lemon juice and zest; mix well. Pour over crust.

5. Bake in the preheated oven for 25 minutes. Cool slightly, then cut into squares while warm; dust with confectioners' sugar.

Prep Time: 10 mins

Total Time: 5 hrs 5 mins

Servings: 8

Ingredients

- 1 tablespoon matcha green tea powder, or more to taste
- 1 cup whole milk
- 2 cups heavy whipping cream
- ¾ cup white sugar
- 2 eggs

Directions

1. Whisk matcha powder in a bowl to remove any lumps; add a splash of milk and whisk until matcha powder is completely dissolved. Gradually whisk remaining milk into matcha mixture.
2. Combine cream and matcha mixture in a pot over medium-low heat; cook, stirring occasionally, until heated through, about 5 minutes.
3. Whisk sugar and eggs together in a bowl. Pour 1/2 cup hot matcha mixture into egg mixture; mix thoroughly. Repeat with remaining matcha mixture. Pour mixture back into the pot.

4. Cook and stir matcha mixture over medium-low heat until heated through, about 3 minutes. Remove from heat and cool to room temperature. Refrigerate until chilled, at least 4 hours.
5. Pour cooled matcha mixture into an ice cream maker and freeze according to the manufacturer's instructions.

Prep Time: 25 mins

Total Time: 1 hr 25 mins

Servings: 24

Ingredients

- ⅓ cup margarine, melted
- ⅔ cup light brown sugar, packed
- 1 pinch salt
- ¾ cup all-purpose flour
- ¼ cup semisweet mini chocolate chips
- 1 (8 ounce) package cream cheese, softened
- 1 (16 ounce) package confectioners' sugar
- 1 cup semisweet mini chocolate chips, melted
- 1 teaspoon vanilla extract

Directions

1. Line a 9x9 inch baking dish with aluminum foil, and set aside.
2. To make the cookie dough pieces, mix the melted margarine, brown sugar, and salt in a bowl. Stir in the flour to make a dough, and knead in 1/4 cup of chocolate chips. Form the dough into a disk about 1/2 inch to 3/4 inch thick, place it on a

sheet of plastic wrap, and then shape the disk into a square with your hands.

3. Place the square piece of dough in the freezer for about 10 minutes, until cold and stiff, and then slice it into 1/2 inch square pieces. Refrigerate the dough pieces while you make the cream cheese fudge.

4. Mix together the cream cheese and confectioners' sugar in a bowl until smooth, and stir in the melted chocolate chips and vanilla extract.

5. Lightly fold in the cookie dough pieces, and spread the candy out into the prepared dish. Refrigerate at least 1 hour, or until firm, and remove the candy from the foil-lined dish. Cut into squares, and serve.

Prep Time: 35 mins

Total Time: 1 hr 15 mins

Servings: 8

Ingredients

- 1 cup peeled, cored, and chopped pears
- ½ cup white sugar
- ½ teaspoon ground ginger
- ¼ teaspoon ground cloves
- ⅓ cup vegetable oil
- 1 teaspoon vanilla extract
- 2 eggs, beaten
- 1 cup all-purpose flour
- 1 teaspoon baking soda
- ¼ teaspoon baking powder
- ½ teaspoon salt

Directions

1. Toss chopped pears with sugar, ginger, and cloves in a large bowl. Set aside and let the sugar dissolve in the pear juices.
2. Preheat oven to 325 degrees F (165 degrees C). Grease an 8x4-inch loaf pan.

3. Stir vegetable oil, vanilla extract, and eggs into the pears. In a separate bowl, combine flour, baking soda, baking powder, and salt. Add the flour mixture to the pear mixture and stir gently just to combine. Pour the batter into the prepared loaf pan.
4. Bake in the preheated oven until golden brown and a toothpick inserted in the center comes out clean, about 40 minutes.

16. Rhubarb Strawberry Crunch

Prep Time: 15 mins
Total Time: 1 hr

Servings: 18

Ingredients

Fruit Layer:

- 3 cups sliced fresh strawberries
- 3 cups diced rhubarb
- 1 cup white sugar
- 3 tablespoons all-purpose flour

Crunch Topping:

- 1 ½ cups all-purpose flour
- 1 cup packed brown sugar
- 1 cup rolled oats
- 1 cup butter

Directions

1. Preheat the oven to 375 degrees F (190 degrees C).
2. Make the fruit layer: Mix strawberries, rhubarb, white sugar, and flour together in a large bowl. Place the mixture in a 9x13-inch baking dish.

3. Make the topping: Combine 1 1/2 cups flour, brown sugar, oats, and butter and mix until crumbly. You may want to use a pastry cutter for this. Sprinkle on top of the rhubarb and strawberry layer.
4. Bake in the preheated oven until crisp and lightly browned, about 45 minutes.

17. Mackerel Dip

Prep Time: 15 mins

Total Time: 2 hrs 15 mins

Servings: 12

Ingredients

- 1 (15 ounce) can mackerel, drained and rinsed
- 1 small onion, finely diced
- ¼ cup tomato-based hot pepper sauce
- 2 teaspoons salt, or to taste
- 1 teaspoon ground black pepper, or to taste
- 1 cup mayonnaise

Directions

1. Remove skin and bones from fish. In a medium bowl, mix fish with onion and hot pepper sauce with a fork, breaking fish into small pieces. Mix in mayonnaise. Season to taste with salt and pepper. Cover, and refrigerate for 2 hours.

18. Delicious Creamed Kale With Mushrooms

Prep Time: 20 mins

Total Time: 35 mins

Servings: 4

Ingredients

- 3 tablespoons butter
- 1 bunch kale, stems removed and leaves chopped
- 1 large shallot, thinly sliced
- 5 crimini mushrooms, sliced
- ¾ cup heavy whipping cream
- ¼ cup shredded Asiago cheese
- 4 cloves garlic, crushed to a paste
- 1 pinch salt and ground black pepper to taste

Directions

1. Heat butter in a large skillet over medium heat; cook and stir kale and shallot until kale is tender, about 5 minutes. Stir mushrooms, cream, Asiago cheese, garlic, salt, and black pepper into kale mixture. Reduce heat to low and simmer until cream has thickened and mushrooms are tender, about 10 minutes.

19. Vegetarian Bolognese with Soy Chorizo

Prep Time: 10 mins

Total Time: 25 mins

Servings: 8

Ingredients

- 3 cups water
- 1 (16 ounce) package thin spaghetti
- 1 tablespoon olive oil
- 18 ounces marinara sauce
- 1 (14.5 ounce) can diced tomatoes
- 12 ounces soy chorizo
- 1 teaspoon dried oregano
- ½ teaspoon cayenne pepper
- ½ teaspoon paprika
- 2 teaspoons chopped fresh basil
- ½ teaspoon freshly ground black pepper

Directions

1. Bring about 3 cups lightly salted water to a boil in a medium-sized pot. Add pasta and cook, stirring occasionally, until tender yet firm to the bite, about 11 minutes.
2. Meanwhile, heat olive oil over medium heat in a large skillet. Add marinara sauce and diced

tomatoes and stir. Add soy chorizo and mix until texture is even, 3 to 5 minutes. Add oregano, cayenne pepper, and paprika; reduce heat and simmer until pasta has finished cooking, about 8 minutes more. Add basil.

3. Drain cooked pasta; top with sauce. Season with black pepper and salt.

20. Ramen Coleslaw

Prep Time: 15 mins

Total Time: 25 mins

Servings: 4

Ingredients

- 2 tablespoons vegetable oil
- 3 tablespoons white wine vinegar
- 2 tablespoons white sugar
- 1 (3 ounce) package chicken flavored ramen noodles, crushed, seasoning packet reserved
- ½ teaspoon salt
- ½ teaspoon ground black pepper
- 2 tablespoons sesame seeds
- ¼ cup sliced almonds
- ½ medium head cabbage, shredded
- 5 green onions, chopped

Directions

1. Preheat oven to 350 degrees F (175 degrees C).
2. In a medium bowl, whisk together the oil, vinegar, sugar, ramen noodle spice mix, salt and pepper to create a dressing.

3. Place sesame seeds and almonds in a single layer on a medium baking sheet. Bake in the preheated oven 10 minutes, or until lightly brown.

4. In a large salad bowl, combine the cabbage, green onions and crushed ramen noodles. Pour dressing over the cabbage, and toss to coat evenly. Top with toasted sesame seeds and almonds.

21. Football Sunday Beer Cheese Soup

Prep Time: 25 mins

Total Time: 45 mins

Servings: 4

Ingredients

- 2 tablespoons butter
- 2 tablespoons minced onion
- 1 teaspoon minced garlic
- 1 ½ tablespoons Worcestershire sauce
- 1 (12 fluid ounce) can or bottle light beer
- 1 ¾ cups chicken broth
- 1 teaspoon ground mustard
- 2 cups half-and-half cream
- 3 cups shredded Cheddar cheese
- ¼ cup flour
- ¼ cup cornstarch
- ¼ cup water

Directions

1. Melt the butter in a saucepan over medium heat; cook the onion and garlic in the butter until the onion is tender, about 5 minutes. Pour in the Worcestershire sauce and beer; bring to a boil for 3 to 5 minutes. Stir the chicken broth and

mustard. Reduce heat to medium-low and pour in the half-and-half while stirring.

2. Toss together the shredded Cheddar cheese and flour in a bowl; add to the liquid mixture in small batches until melted.

3. Whisk together the cornstarch and warm water in a small bowl; stir into the cheese mixture; season with salt and pepper. Heat and stir until thick; serve hot.

Prep Time: 5 mins

Total Time: 5 mins

Servings: 1

Ingredients

- 1 ½ fluid ounces vodka
- 4 fluid ounces cranberry juice
- 1 fluid ounce grapefruit juice
- 1 ½ cups ice cubes
- 1 lime wedge

Directions

1. Combine vodka, cranberry juice, and grapefruit juice in a highball glass and stir to combine. Add ice.
2. Garnish with a wedge of lime.

23. Oatmeal Banana Nut Cookies

Prep Time: 30 mins

Total Time: 30 mins

Servings: 18

Ingredients

- 1 cup butter
- 1 cup white sugar
- 1 cup packed brown sugar
- 2 eggs
- 1 teaspoon banana extract
- 1 ½ cups all-purpose flour
- 1 teaspoon baking soda
- ½ teaspoon salt
- 3 cups rolled oats
- 2 cups chopped pecans

Directions

1. Preheat oven to 375 degrees F (190 degrees C).
2. Cream butter or margarine with mixer. Blend in whole eggs, sugar, and extract. Add flour, baking soda, and salt. When the ingredients are thoroughly mixed, add oats and pecans. Mix on lower speed until consistent.

3. Drop pieces of the dough using an ice cream scoop onto an ungreased cookie tray roughly 3 to 4 inches apart.
4. Bake 8 to 10 minutes. Eight minutes would yield crispy cookies with a chewy, slightly doughy center. For harder, crispier cookies, bake longer. Cool on wire rac

24. Easy Shrimp Mozambique

Prep Time: 15 mins

Total Time: 30 mins

Servings: 4

Ingredients

- 4 tablespoons butter
- ¼ cup finely chopped onion
- ½ cup water
- 1 lemon, juiced
- 8 cloves garlic, finely chopped
- 2 (1.41 ounce) packages sazon seasoning with saffron salt and ground black pepper to taste
- ½ (12 ounce) bottle beer
- 2 teaspoons hot sauce or to taste
- 1 pound uncooked medium shrimp, peeled and deveined

Directions

1. Melt butter in a saucepan over medium heat. Add onion and saute until slightly golden, about 5 minutes. Stir in water, lemon juice, garlic, sazon, salt, and pepper. Cook for 2 minutes. Pour in beer and stir. Add hot sauce; bring to a boil. Add shrimp and cook until pink, about 3 minutes.

25. Frangipane Pear Tart

Prep Time: 30 mins

Total Time: 2 hrs 15 mins

Servings: 8

Ingredients

Pears:

- 4 cups water
- 1 cup white sugar
- 2 tablespoons honey
- 1 vanilla bean, split lengthwise
- 1 cinnamon stick
- 5 pods cardamom, crushed
- 4 Conference pears - peeled, halved, and cored

Pastry:

- 1 ½ cups all-purpose flour
- ½ cup confectioners' sugar
- ½ teaspoon salt
- ½ cup cold unsalted butter, cut into pieces
- 1 tablespoon cold unsalted butter, cut into pieces
- 1 egg yolk

Frangipane:

- ⅔ cup white sugar

- ⅓ cup unsalted butter, at room temperature
- ¾ cup ground blanched almonds
- 1 egg
- 1 egg white
- 2 teaspoons all-purpose flour
- 1 teaspoon cornstarch
- 2 teaspoons almond extract
- 1 teaspoon vanilla extract

Directions

1. Combine water, 1 cup white sugar, honey, vanilla bean, cinnamon stick, and cardamom in a large saucepan. Bring to a simmer over medium heat. Add pears; reduce heat and simmer until pears are translucent or easily pierced with a knife, about 10 minutes. Remove from heat and cool to room temperature.
2. Combine 1 1/2 cup flour, confectioners' sugar, and salt in a bowl. Cut in 1/2 cup plus 1 tablespoon butter until mixture is crumbly. Mix in egg yolk until dough sticks together in large clumps.
3. Grease a 9-inch tart pan with a removable bottom. Press dough evenly into the pan. Freeze for 30 minutes. Reserve leftover dough for patching cracks.

4. Preheat oven to 375 degrees F (190 degrees C).

5. Grease the shiny side of a piece of aluminum foil with butter; place butter-side down over the pastry. Transfer tart pan to a baking sheet.

6. Bake in the preheated oven, using leftover dough to patch any cracks, until dough looks dry and light brown, about 20 minutes. Peel off aluminum foil; let pastry cool.

7. Reduce oven temperature to 350 degrees F (175 degrees C).

8. Combine 2/3 cup white sugar and 1/3 cup butter in a large bowl; beat with an electric mixer until light and fluffy. Mix in ground almonds. Add egg, egg yolk, 2 teaspoons flour, and cornstarch; beat until frangipane is smooth. Beat in almond extract and vanilla extract.

9. Spread frangipane evenly over the pastry. Drain pear halves and dry with paper towels. Cut lengthwise into even slices. Place 1 pear half on a spatula and gently fan out slices. Place on frangipane. Repeat with remaining pear halvesBake in the preheated oven until frangipane is firm to the touch, 40 to 45 minutes. Cool on a wire rack.

Prep Time: 20 mins

Total Time: 10 hrs 50 mins

Servings: 18

Ingredients

Soaking Syrup:

- 3 cups white sugar
- 2 cups water
- 3 1/4-inch-thick slices peeled fresh ginger
- ½ lemon, zested in large strips
- 1 teaspoon lemon juice

Koeksisters:

- 2 cups cake flour
- 1 tablespoon baking powder
- ¼ teaspoon salt
- 2 tablespoons cold unsalted butter, cut into chunks
- ½ cup milk
- 2 cups oil, or as needed

Directions

1. Combine sugar, water, ginger, lemon zest, and lemon juice together in a saucepan; bring to a

boil, reduce heat to medium, and cook for 10 minutes. Cool syrup to room temperature, transfer to a container, and refrigerate until flavors blend, 8 hours to overnight.

2. Sift flour, baking powder, and salt together in a bowl. Rub the butter into the flour mixture with your fingertips until mixture has a cornmeal texture. Add the milk; mix until a smooth dough forms. Wrap the dough in plastic wrap and let it rest for 2 hours.

3. Turn the dough out onto a lightly floured work surface and roll into a 5x14-inch rectangle about 1/4-inch thick. Cut the dough into twenty eight 1/2-inch wide strips. Twist pairs of strips together and pinch the ends together. Repeat for all of the strips. Cover strips with a clean cloth and let rest for 15 minutes.

4. Heat about 2-inches of oil in a deep-fryer or large saucepan to 350 degrees F (175 degrees C). Place a wire rack over a baking sheet.

5. Pour some of the cold syrup into a bowl and return remaining syrup to the refrigerator.

6. Working in batches, fry koeksister twists in hot oil until twists swell and are golden brown, 2 to 5 minutes. Remove koeksisters from hot oil with a slotted spoon and immediately immerse in cold syrup for 10 seconds. Transfer soaked koeksisters to prepared wire rack to cool. Replenish cold syrup as necessary.

27. Spicy Lime Grilled Shrimp

Prep Time: 5 mins

Total Time: 30 mins

Servings: 8

Ingredients

- 3 tablespoons Cajun seasoning
- 1 lime, juiced
- 1 tablespoon vegetable oil
- 1 pound peeled and deveined medium shrimp (30-40 per pound)

Directions

1. Mix together the Cajun seasoning, lime juice, and vegetable oil in a resealable plastic bag. Add the shrimp, coat with the marinade, squeeze out excess air, and seal the bag. Marinate in the refrigerator for 20 minutes.
2. Preheat an outdoor grill for medium heat, and lightly oil the grate. Remove the shrimp from the marinade, and shake off excess. Discard the remaining marinade.
3. Cook the shrimp on the preheated grill until they are bright pink on the outside and the meat is no

longer transparent in the center, about 2 minutes per side.

28. Lola's Horchata

Prep Time: 10 mins

Total Time: 3 h

Servings: 3

Ingredients

- 5 cups water
- 1 cup uncooked white long-grain rice
- ⅔ cup white sugar
- ½ cup milk
- ½ tablespoon vanilla extract
- ½ tablespoon ground cinnamon

Directions

1. Pour water and rice into a blender; mix until rice begins to break up, about 1 minute. Let rice and water stand at room temperature for at least 3 hours.
2. Strain rice water into a pitcher and discard rice. Stir in sugar, milk, vanilla, and cinnamon.
3. Chill thoroughly before serving over ice.

29. Pangalactic Gargleblaster

Prep Time: 5 mins

Total Time: 5 mins

Servings: 1

Ingredients

- 1 tablespoon gin
- 1 tablespoon light rum
- 1 tablespoon vodka
- 1 tablespoon tequila
- 2 tablespoons creme de menthe liqueur
- 2 tablespoons Galliano
- 1 cup ice cubes
- 1 slice lemon

Directions

1. Combine the gin, rum, vodka, tequila, creme de menthe, Galliano and ice in the container of a blender. Cover, and blend until slushy. Pour into a glass and garnish with a slice of lemon.

30. Tomato Chicken Parmesan

Prep Time: 15 mins

Total Time: 45 mins

Servings: 6

Ingredients

- 2 eggs, beaten
- 1 cup grated Parmesan cheese
- 7 ounces seasoned bread crumbs
- 6 skinless, boneless chicken breast halves
- 1 tablespoon vegetable oil
- 12 ounces pasta sauce
- 6 slices Monterey Jack cheese

Directions

1. Preheat oven to 375 degrees F (190 degrees C).
2. Pour beaten eggs into a shallow dish or bowl. In another shallow dish or bowl, mix together the grated Parmesan cheese and bread crumbs. Dip chicken breasts into beaten egg, then into bread crumb mixture to coat.
3. In a large skillet, heat oil over medium high heat. Add coated chicken and saute for about 8 to 10 minutes each side, or until chicken is cooked through and juices run clear.

4. Pour tomato sauce into a lightly greased 9x13 inch baking dish. Add chicken, then place a slice of Monterey Jack cheese over each breast, and bake in the preheated oven for 20 minutes or until cheese is completely melted.

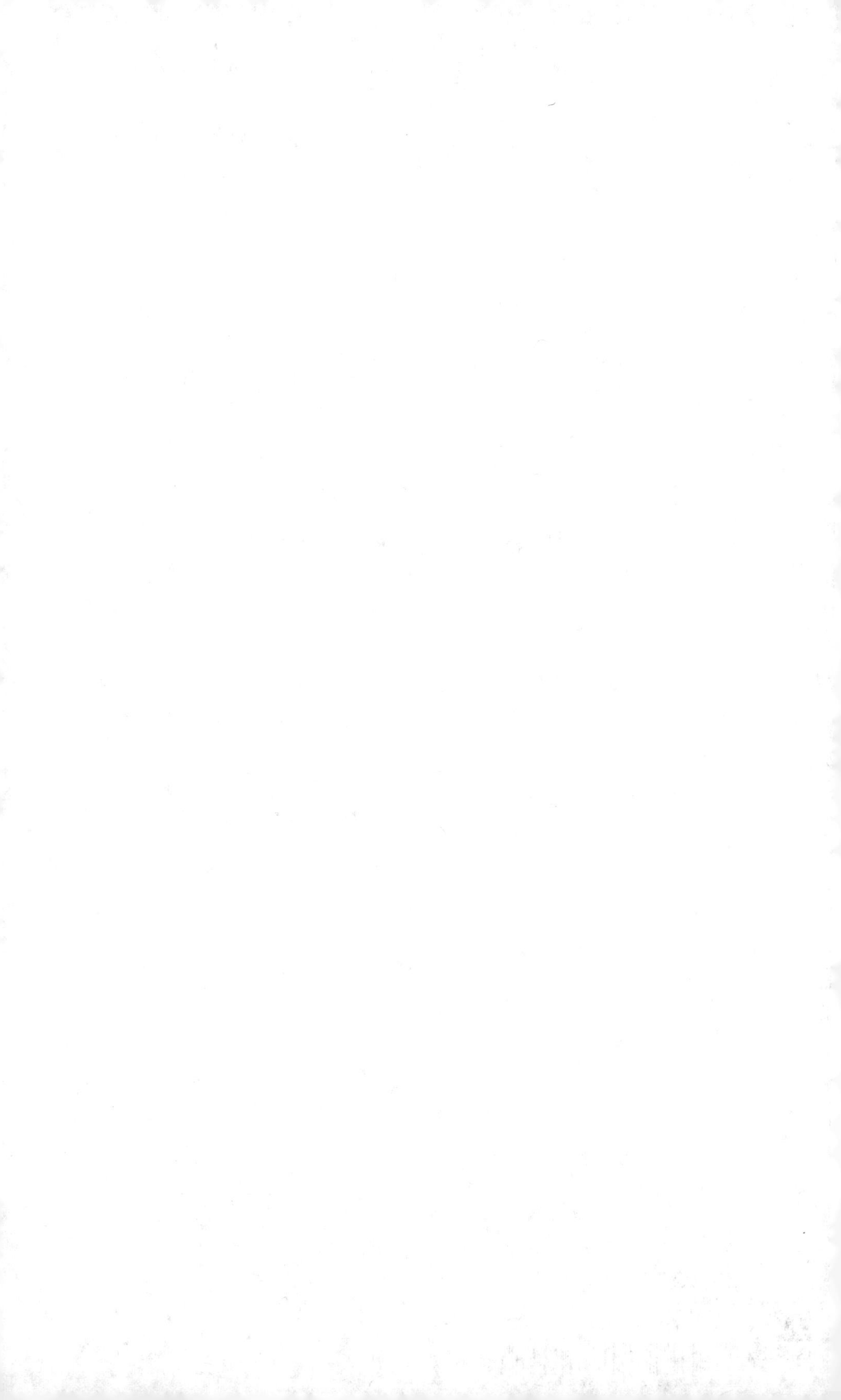